CALMING THE EMOTIONAL STORM OF BREAST CANCER

Tess Taft, MSW, LICSW
Kathy Beach, RN
Christopher M. Lee, MD

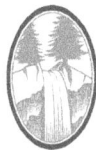

PROVENIR PUBLISHING
Spokane, Washington

www.provenirpublishing.com

Calming The Emotional Storm Of Breast Cancer

Published by Provenir Publishing, LLC, P. O. Box 211, Greenacres, WA 99016-0211

Production Credits

Lead Editor: Christopher Lee

Production Director: Amy Hanson

Art Director and Illustration: Micah Harman

Cover Photo: Micah Harman

Printing History: May 2013, First Edition.

This book is dedicated to our patients and their families,
who inspire us every day in their cancer fight.

For most patients, the words "you have breast cancer" are some of the most stressful that they have ever heard. In addition to being stressful for the person with the diagnosis, this can also be a challenging time for their family members, close friends, and loved ones. The diagnosis of one person can have a wide and lasting effect on many people.

Most care providers know that it is impossible for anyone to face a breast cancer diagnosis and not have major stress added to their life and the lives of everyone who loves them. In fact, many patients state that cancer is the most difficult challenge they have ever faced. In addition to the added stress of the diagnosis, the standard cancer therapies and treatments can also be difficult and require great inner strength, perseverance, and resolve. Because of this, a strong support group of friends and family can provide great relief and can become a life-line.

This handbook was written to empower those of you struggling with breast cancer, and your loved ones, with stress management tools to support you during your difficult journey from diagnosis through treatment and beyond. It was written by Tess Taft, an oncology family therapist and stress management specialist, who has many years of experience counseling patients and families who are navigating their way through the dark night of breast cancer treatment. Although each person's background and situation is different, we trust these tools can provide assistance to you and your loved ones during this life changing time.

Chapter One

Calming The Emotional Storm Of Breast Cancer

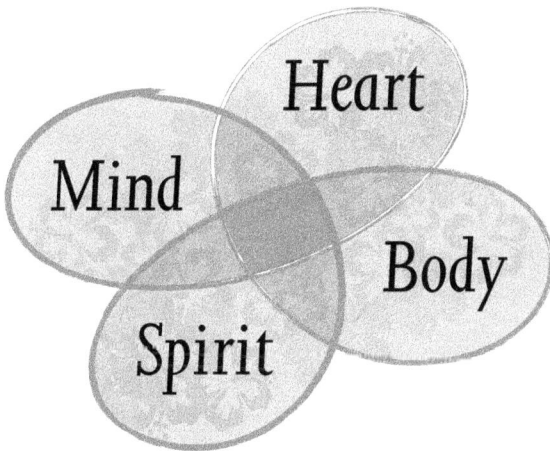

Calming The Emotional Storm

A diagnosis of breast cancer is a crisis large enough to impact your body, your mind, your heart, and your spirit. Breast cancer is a family disease because it affects everyone you love, and in different ways. Today women and men with breast cancer are living longer and healthier lives than ever before. Even so, it remains a large enough crisis to change your life immediately in ways that cause you to suffer, and in other more positive ways you won't recognize until later, perhaps much later. You have a lot of work ahead as you face treatment and living with a chronic disease, as breast cancer is understood today. You will feel discouraged and then find your strength and resilience over and over. If you think about it, curing and healing are different. The work of your physicians is to find a cure, or ways to prolong your life. You have an equally important job. Your job is to find ways and people who can help you heal the emotional and spiritual suffering generated by breast cancer, and to allow cancer to become your teacher. To be able to manage your new and different life you must learn to truly live, grow, express your own needs, and have your own back.

Chapter Two

Focusing On Your Body

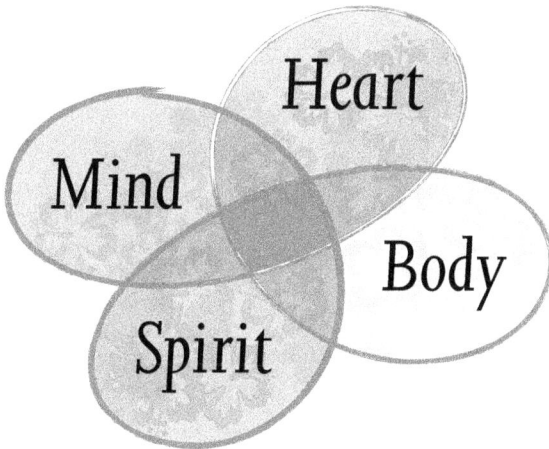

Heart

Mind

Body

Spirit

Your Physical Experience

"Why does the smallest part of me give me the most trouble?!"

"I blamed myself for this. Nobody in my family has had it. I thought I got this because I didn't take good care of my body. I never learned how to manage my stress. I finally stopped hating my- self when my doctor asked me this: 'Where do you want your focus to be--on blaming yourself or on healing?' I had to choose, since I couldn't focus on both. I chose healing."

"I bought some beautiful camisoles. I need to hide from his eyes for awhile."

"I feel guilty. I've worked since I was 16. The rest of society is working. Am I being lazy taking time off for treatment?"

"You'll hear me say 'I haven't got the energy'. But please keep asking me anyway."

"It takes a lot to preserve my dignity and my sense of myself now. I'm tired all of the time."

"I had no idea what the cost of this journey would be when I started treatment. I'd still do it, and fight to live, but I couldn't understand at the beginning."

"I wish I'd had more information about the side effects of radiation before I had them. Maybe somebody told me, but I was surprised and scared. I needed them written out in real language, not medicalese."

"I have friends who have had breast cancer. They smile and as-sure me I can do the treatment, all of it. They are so encouraging. I don't know what I'd do without them."

"Is this the best I'm going to feel? I might be taking treatment for years. I can't do what I used to do, like hike in the mountains. If this is as good as it's going to get, what makes my life worth living?"

Tips For The Journey:

Remember that your whole body is not sick, although it may feel like that. Aside from the cancer, how well is your body working for you now? Some people feel more hopeful when they remember that in general their body is doing well, in spite of the cancer.

Think about all the ways your body has stood by you in the past, the times you've been ill and recovered, the times your body has responded well to medical interventions, the ways your body has told you what it needs and how you have responded. You're simply doing that again, even with the cancer. Your body knows how to heal.

Respect the needs of your body as you move through treatment. Many people with breast cancer feel exhausted by treatment. You will need more rest than you think. Don't push your body, which is working so hard to absorb and process different medications and procedures while maintaining normal functioning at the same time. Your body is working overtime to get you well again and to heal, which requires enormous energy. Lovingly, give it a break.

It's important to bring someone with you to doctor appointments and chemo sessions. This needs to be someone you don't have to take care of, or entertain, or even talk to. Choose someone who can just sit and be with you, who can be another listening ear when your medical team gives you information. Research shows that people hear about 30% of the information presented to them when they are stressed, not to mention when chemo brain (the temporary, short term memory loss associated with chemotherapy) complicates memory and communication.

After surgery, husbands or partners can feel pressured to tell you that you look fine, when they may not initially feel that way. If you are heading into surgery, close your eyes for a moment and imagine surgery is complete and has gone very well, and the bandages are being removed. With your mind's eye, look down where your breast was and imagine what you see. What is your very first reaction? Can you give your husband or partner the gift of the same first reaction you imagine yourself feeling?

Whether or not you decide to have reconstructive surgery, you will experience a period of time when you are adjusting to your new appearance. Many women have ambivalent feelings about the surgery; they are grateful to be alive, to have the obvious cancer removed, but dislike how they look or

Nurse's Note:

Some people like to journal during treatment. This can help them clarify and express their feelings.

5

feel. This can be especially true for women whose breasts are a crucial part of their sexuality or key to feeling like a woman. Allow yourself to take the time you need to come to terms privately with your "new" breast or breasts. Allow yourself to grieve. Talk about your feelings with your partner. Women often assume the change will be very upsetting to their partners, when in fact they will come to terms with the loss just as you will. A breast cancer support group can be a big help at this time, since women who have been in the group for awhile are often comfortable showing newcomers their own reconstructed breasts. Having no reconstruction is also an option many women are most comfortable with. Some women like their reconstructed breasts better than the originals. Over time you will come to terms with your new look, and gratitude for health will outweigh your doubts about how your breasts look or feel.

Prioritize the precious energy you have. Decide what you want to do, then pace yourself so that you can avoid "crashing" into exhaustion and the misery that comes with it. Is completing a task most important, so that you can feel useful? Is it sharing time with a loved one that will fill your need today? Make a list of what you'd like to do. Choose. You probably can't do everything on your list, so trim it in order to stay focused on what you can do, instead of what you can't. If you choose to do more than your level of energy can handle, schedule time to rest so your body can get back to healing. You'll feel more in control and content.

Ask the people who love you for some ideas of things you can do that don't require physical effort. If chemo brain is holding you captive, ask for ideas for movies you might like. Funny movies are good for your immune system. War like films might inspire the fight in you. Books with short stories or stories of how others with cancer have coped, healed or gained wisdom can help. Meet your own needs.

Allow people to help you. Be specific in your requests. People with cancer say that it's much harder to receive than to give, but remember: you are giving people a gift by receiving their help. They feel helpless, and any ways they are allowed to be helpful to you helps them, too. They're a part of your team. Relinquish thoughts that you can handle this journey alone, or that your family can manage it alone. When friends ask what they can do to help, ask one of them to organize a work party for you. Have a good friend make up the work list. Your job is to join them by doing the least demanding job on the list, or to sit back and rest, feeling loved and cared for.

The goal is not to endure stress, but to manage it. Receiving help is a management skill.

Reduce the physical challenges of treatment by finding ways to help yourself relax. Feeling the need to be constantly alert, ready for battle, sword in hand, is common among people facing a life-threatening disease. It can help prevent more bad news from being the kind of shock you felt at your first diagnosis. But the need to relax during your cancer journey is crucial for your healing, and the price of remaining hyper-vigilant is always feeling the threat of more cancer hanging over your head. Letting go for awhile with a hot bath, yoga, relaxation exercises, guided imagery, massage, meditation or prayer will help strengthen your immune system, your mood, and your ability to bring new energy to the fight.

Perhaps most important of all, remember that you are not the disease. You are not the problem. Cancer is. You are much more than the cancer. You are a person who is loved and valued, well or sick, vital or exhausted.

Chapter Three

Focusing On Your Mind

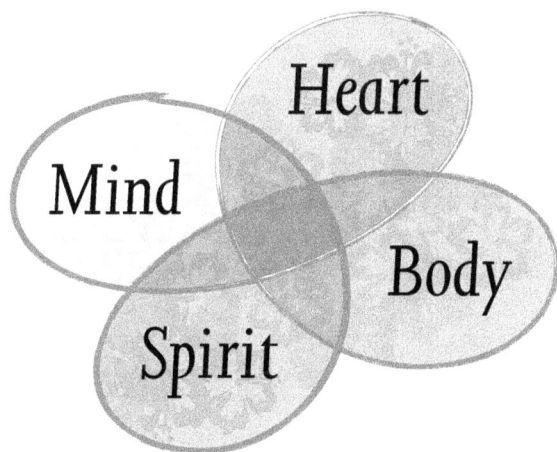

Heart

Mind

Body

Spirit

Your Thoughts And Beliefs About Cancer

"My doctor said something that really helped. He said 'Don't pay any attention to statistics or anecdotal information. It's your cancer, not anybody else's.'"

"Cancer is not my diagnosis—it's our diagnosis. I want to protect my whole family from being scared, but it's really hard to protect them from my fears and communicate well at the same time. I keep biting my tongue."

"I heard the word cancer and I didn't hear another thing. I feel like I can't even think. All I can do is feel, and feel scared."

"I'm terrified most of the time. I try not to listen to everything people say so I can stay focused on today and the next step I have to take."

"Some of my friends can't come with me into my cancer world. They keep talking about my reconstructive surgery when I'll be 'back to normal again'. But I'll never be the same person I used to be. What if they don't like me then? What if I don't feel close to them?"

"The life I knew is gone. It's over. My goal was to get to 70 years old without taking any meds. I was an icon of health. I have to learn to think differently about my health now."

"Everybody has ideas of what I should do and how I should handle this, and I don't know who to listen to."

"I'm the 'caregiver' I read about. I'm her husband. She's always asked how she's doing. People don't ask me that. Why not? I'm overwhelmed."

She: "I don't talk about pain. I don't want to explain it all the time. I don't care about the broken dishwasher!"

He: "When she's in pain or tired she's short tempered, grumpy and she barks at me. I need to not take it personally."

"I have to ask people to help me. That's easier to do now that I'm not so angry at the world for my getting cancer."

"I just deny that I could die. I don't even think about it. Is something wrong with me?"

"I had to change my whole perception of my cancer. I finally allowed myself to be ill. I accepted my illness, and then I could let go of so much suffering."

"I'm the key member of my medical team here. I'm the key decision maker."

"Go ahead and change doctors if you don't feel you 'click' with the doctor you have, or if you're not getting your questions answered. Do you wonder what chemo is like? Or radiation? Ask! This is your life you're fighting for!"

"The scheduler told me 'We can't get you in for two weeks' and I freaked. I wanted to yell 'Don't you understand? I'm dying of cancer here!' That was 4 years ago. I'm so thankful that urgency is gone."

"I feel limited by my own thinking. I don't want to plan things. If I leave town and something goes wrong, what would I do?"

"I'm done with treatment. Am I done with cancer? How can I stay well by myself?"

"I felt the need to do the paperwork—you know, the end of life decisions—so that when I die nobody has to deal with all of that. My family was horrified that I found it comforting."

"I was the rock in the family. I knew what everyone should do and how to do it. I can't do that any more. They need to be their own rock and use their own best judgment from now on."

Tips For The Journey:

For many there is an urge to stay silent in order to protect loved ones from powerful fears and anger, and an equally strong need to talk. Find someone you can be totally honest with, who can listen without giving advice or opinions. Allow yourself to express your fears fully so that you can let them go for now. This might be someone in your family or it might be a trusted friend. You can contact a cancer support group in your area. These are the people who really get it, since they are dealing with some of the same issues themselves. You can seek the loving ear of a spiritual advisor or a psychotherapist. Be wary of internet chat rooms and

Nurse's Note:

Don't hesitate to let your caregivers know how you are feeling. They are there to help you.

blogs. Many people become more frightened while exploring because they are exposed to other peoples' fears.

Just as you need the freedom and space to express your feelings, so do your children or grandchildren. Your cancer center may offer (or be willing to start) a national project of the Annie E. Casey Foundation called Kidz Count, which welcomes children whose parent or grandparent has cancer. Without this program, many children feel alone and unable to find the words or support from peers to help with the feelings that haunt them.

Many couples, when one partner is diagnosed with cancer, try to protect the other from their deep fears and concerns, and choose not to talk about how they are really doing. This can cause an invisible wall to descent between you, making you feel like friendly roommates instead of intimate partners. It can become harder and harder to talk honestly when this happens. Some people find themselves having the most personal conversations only with someone other than their partner, which, over time, can cause damage to the relationship. Go ahead and cry together, talk together, listen to each other's fears, and comfort each other. Get some couples counseling if you need it; this is a time of crisis. You'll feel less alone and you'll know that you're part of a team facing the cancer together. This, over time, will strengthen your relationship. Join a cancer support group together, or look for a caregiver support group in your area so your spouse or partner can get help with feelings of isolation, frustration, fear and guilt so common to these special people whose world has turned upside down as well. Many religious organizations, the Quakers and Mormons among them, form a care committee to organize help when anyone among them is sick or disabled. You can do this, too.

Couples can find it helpful to talk about their relationship when one of them becomes ill. Every couple has made agreements, spoken and unspoken, about how they will be with each other. A wedding vow is such a contract. It can be helpful to clarify the unspoken assumptions you each hold about illness, what caring for each other means during illness, and what it means to give and receive support.

Be aware that some of your friends may appear to withdraw from you when they discover you have cancer. You may be thinking "When you get cancer you sure find out who your friends are". The truth is that they don't know what to say to you, or they are afraid they will cry in your presence, adding the burden of their fears or grief to your load. The longer this estrangement goes on, the guiltier they feel. Instead of feeling abandoned you could choose to initiate contact with them and let them know you miss them and would welcome their presence, in a real way, at this time.

On the other hand, there may be friends who you'd rather not be in contact with now. When you're with them you may feel their needs weighing you down, or that you need to use precious energy to attend to them. You may simply want to avoid the ubiquitous question, "How ARE you?", asked with deep concern. An option is to go online to sites such as Caring Bridge or Helping Hands, where you can enter information and updates you're comfortable sharing that others can access. This will give you more privacy and prevent you from having to answer the same questions over and over. Friends and acquaintances can send you messages this way, too.

Most people fighting cancer hear intense and heartfelt advice about which doctors to see and which alternative or complementary treatments to try. Some can be very insistent. This can be very confusing and frightening. If this kind of talk is not helpful, you can respond by saying, "Thanks for your thoughts and for caring about me, but I trust the doctors I'm working with and I'm not looking for other treatments right now. I'll let you know if I change my mind." If you are interested in finding an oncology naturopath to complement your medical treatment, look online. You may be able to consult on the phone if the doctor is located at a distance. Most important of all, trust the carefully considered decisions you, your loved ones and your doctors have chosen to help you heal.

Sometimes people say they're coping by being in denial. They are simply pacing themselves, accepting information at a speed they can tolerate as time goes by. From diagnosis through treatment, cancer is a long haul.

People with cancer are often approached by friends and coworkers who, for some reason, feel free to share the most horrifying, tragic stories of cancer suffering they know. Be prepared. You'll hear stories about relatives, friends, friends of friends, and strangers and all of the ways they suffered. Allow yourself to immediately interrupt these stories, saying something like, "That story makes me feel nervous, uncomfortable, bad, or _____. Let's talk about something else."

When treatment is done a new set of challenges appear. There is no going "back to normal". There is only moving forward, creating a "new normal" life. You will find yourself relaxing into your new life if you take the time to deeply consider what you've been left with after cancer, what you've been gifted with by the cancer, what you choose to bring into your life now, and what you choose to leave behind. One thing that stays is this: you will wonder if cancer will come back and kill you until you die of something else. You can make this decision: "If I have to deal with cancer again, I will."

Chapter Four

Focusing On Your Heart

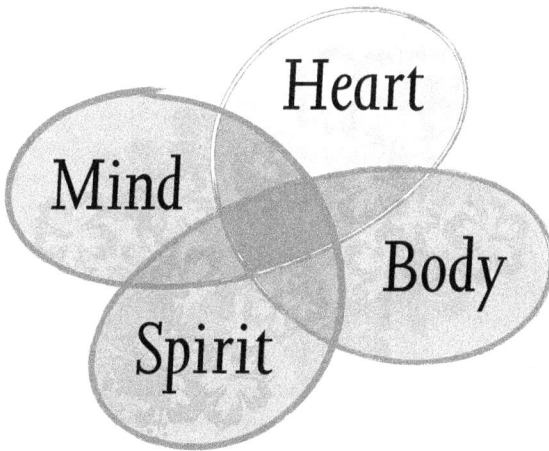

Heart

Mind

Body

Spirit

The Ways You Feel About Yourself, Your Life, And Cancer

"I'm so scared all the time. I've heard so many awful things about treatment. Poison, slash and burn. How will I survive this? Some days all I want to do is walk away from it all."

"I got the shovel out again today. I'm digging my own grave. I've got to get a handle on my anxiety."

"My three year old saw a bald mannequin in a store and yelled 'Look Mommy! She's bald, just like you!' I can't hide my cancer, even with this great wig."

"I hate my body. I hate how it feels. I hate the scars. I hate my breast being gone. My whole body is way off. It's not me."

"Why don't I feel anything? What's wrong with me?"

"I know I have to keep a positive attitude or I'll die."

"If my test comes back bad, I'm screwed. If it comes back with good news, I still worry."

"I have anxiety, but I'm slowing my pace as I race to the edge of the cliff. My life doesn't feel like it's going to explode the way it did when I got diagnosed. Everything I worry about doesn't need to be weighed so heavily. I'm finding my balance."

"I feel so useless when I don't have any energy. I always took charge. I was the one people depended on. I just can't be that person now. I feel like such a burden on my family."

"I get so scared about my medical care sometimes. If I'm un-happy with something they say or do, and I'm not nice, will they give up on me or not try so hard to save my life? I finally asked my doctor that and she was amazed. She wanted to know when I wasn't happy. So make sure you ask your questions, and insist on answers in ways you understand. It will give you a sense of control."

"How will my having no breasts affect my husband in the long run? Now he's OK with it, but what about 5 years from now? Will he want to have an affair?"

"I thought my husband wasn't attracted to me during treatment, but it was me that I wasn't attracted to."

"I'm done tormenting myself about how I look now. I'm done."

"When my wife was diagnosed, my first thought was 'Everybody knows it's a death sentence. She's going to die.' For the first six months there was so much fear and anger. My brain was consumed with thoughts of cancer and treatment and survival. Now, four and a half years into it, here we are, happier than we've ever been. I'm not raging at the world. Our focus is on today, on right now. We watch birds eating mountain ash berries. Did you know some birds eat them whole and others eat only the insides?"

"I'm finally mad about what cancer has done to the life I had."

"I'm beginning to understand that I deserve all the help I'm getting. It's a big step from feeling desperate, like I had to have it but was putting everyone out. I deserve it. Isn't that amazing?"

"I'm a man with breast cancer. Try telling that to your friends. It's embarrassing. I don't want to talk about it."

"My family and friends can get a break from the cancer by withdrawing from me for awhile. I can never get a break."

"I just can't bring myself to discipline the kids any more. In case I die, I don't want to leave them with bad memories. It drives my husband crazy."

"I do the cancer stomp dance with my kids when any of us gets scared. We laugh. It helps."

"If I relax and put the fear down, the cancer will sneak up on me again. I never want to feel that shock of being diagnosed with cancer again."

"When I'm depressed I go somewhere else. I stop. I freeze in place and quit taking care of myself."

"I don't feel whole any more. I want the lives my friends are living."

"Losing my hair felt like one more insult. My cancer became public. I was so embarrassed. I had to become willing to just let myself be embarrassed, but in a softer way. It's not my fault this happened."

"Sex? What's that?"

"Is it depression or is it grief? I think it's grief. I've lost so much."

"What's the hardest loss for me, even though I've been told there's no more evidence of cancer? I'll always wonder if it will come back and kill me. I've lost forever the assumption that I'll die of old age."

"I was sexually assaulted when I was younger. I look at where my breast used to be and feel the way I felt then all over again. I feel like the abuse will never end."

"I long for the carefree days I didn't even know were carefree."

"I'm done with treatment. When am I going to feel like 'YIP-PEE! I DID IT!'?"

"I'm done with treatment. I actually feel good. My husband and family are absolutely convinced I'm fine again. They can't grieve with me. I don't think I'll ever be done with cancer. I'm in a new world again and I don't understand this one, either. "

"Breast cancer is so life changing. Now that treatment is done it's still life changing because I don't know how to really live without the routines of treatment, which were so reassuring. My hand was held all the way along. Smart people really had me covered. Now where am I? Who am I? I feel alone with my fears that it will come back. I've made the tamoxifen my routine now, my big morning ritual. My husband thinks I'm nuts."

"Since treatment I'm realizing that we can help our bodies, but we really can't control them. I can hold this truth now without so much pain. It's just life. It moves on. It's all OK, in the long run."

"I wouldn't trade what I've learned from cancer for anything. I was always running in my life. I'm sitting in my life now. I've learned how to replace the old, constant judgment with compassion and respect for myself. That is the gift cancer gave to me. Or maybe

I gave it to myself. "

"*In nature time is so different. It slows down. Don't tie time to a clock. Who knows how long any of us will live?*"

"*I have regrets. I have not lived my life very fully. I've made compromises I wish I hadn't, trying to meet other people's expectations. Cancer changed that. I'm a lot happier with myself now.*"

"*I want to leave a legacy of good work. I may need to leave my work unfinished, unresolved. That breaks my heart.*"

"*When I was first diagnosed I was so stressed I felt close to suicide. I didn't want to hurt anybody, but I just wanted to feel some peace. Then, after a couple of treatments I thought 'OK, I can do this.' I felt much more relaxed. Now, after several years, I don't think about cancer. I think instead about each day. I focus on one day, one symptom at a time.*"

"*I'm learning to check inside and ask myself 'What is the truth here and what is the fear?' I try to separate them now.*"

"*Imagining dying is easier than imagining being happy again.*"

He: "*It's not about her dying somewhere down the road. It's about loving her now. Worrying about her dying is wasting precious time. To people just hearing they have breast cancer, or any cancer, I'd say 'You will get to a place where you know this and are more at peace. I promise.*"

Tips For The Journey:

It will help if you think back on the hardest times you have already survived in your life. How did you make it through? What coping skills did you depend on? Did you need to talk, or withdraw for awhile? Did you allow yourself to feel sad, or angry? Did gathering information help? Did you need to turn the whole thing over to the "professionals" to "fix" so that you could relax? Did you have ways to distract yourself when you needed that? Did you pray? Did you allow people who loved you to help you? How? What worked back then? Tell a trusted friend the stories of how life has taught you these skills.

Think about the strengths of character you bring to this challenge. Recognize your wisdom, your inner power, your determination. What qualities did you bring to the critical times you've already survived in your life? If you're not sure, ask people who love you. They often see us more clearly than we see ourselves, especially when we are anxious. And, again, tell the stories of how life taught you to find these strengths within yourself.

There is a difference between grief and depression. When we grieve we know exactly why we feel so low. When we are depressed we often live in a cloud of unease and sadness without really knowing why. Sometimes people feel both. Things that used to bring you pleasure, or even deep joy, may feel empty now. Grieve through the losses that diagnosis and treatment have forced upon you. Meetings with a counselor can help you figure out where you are stuck, ways that might help you feel more centered and peaceful, and whether an anti-depressant would help for the time being.

Conflict often happens in families when differing ways of coping with the cancer collide. It is important to allow people to cope in their own ways. For example, one person may be devastated by fears that you will die. Another may be totally focused on what you need to do to complete treatment. Or, one person, in order to relax, may need to hear every update, attend all of your doctor appointments and treatment sessions. For others, this might cause unbearable stress. The statements to avoid among family members are: "You shouldn't feel that way" and "If you love ___ (the person with cancer) enough you'd ___".

Men and women can have different ways of feeling and coping with breast cancer. Men often feel helpless because they can't fix the women they love, and work hard to get life back to "normal" as quickly as possible. Women partners can feel as though he doesn't understand or welcome their need to express fear, sadness and anger. It helps if women can find a breast cancer support group and close friends who can listen. It helps the relationship if both partners can understand and accept that men may not always be able to accompany their partners on the emotional journey of breast cancer.

It is normal to feel very frightened when breast cancer is diagnosed. It is also normal for emotions to sink below awareness at diagnosis. In a crisis we must stay focused. However, don't be surprised later when the feelings of crisis have passed (which they will) and your feelings from diagnosis rise to the surface. If this happens, remember that your emotions are simply catching up with the rest of you. Let yourself express them with someone you trust who can simply listen without having to "fix" you.

Remember this: you are not the burden weighing on the people who love you. The cancer is burdening all of you. For every family, when cancer is diagnosed, the fear of death is real, painful, and lasting. This is called anticipatory grief and it happens when any loved one's life is threatened, whether they die from the disease or not. That is part of the burden cancer places on all of you. Ask someone close to you to remind you of this, that you are not the burden, when you forget it. Most people do.

Children around the age of five (and older) always wonder if their parent is going to die from the cancer. Many of them will come right out and ask, while others hold this secret dread deep inside, causing physical symptoms or fears of going to school and leaving you alone at home. Children also wonder if they caused your cancer. This is what your children need from you: to know that they are loved and will be cared for by someone they trust during those times when you can't. They need to continue their normal routines such as music lessons and sports practices and games. The family rules, like bedtimes, time spent on computer games, etc. need to be maintained as closely as possible. Your children need to hear these promises from you: "I promise that the cancer is not your fault. I promise that I will tell you if I'm going to die from the cancer. Dying is not something the doctors are worried about at all now. So you don't need to worry about it. I want you to promise in exchange that you will come and talk with me when you are scared about this or anything else. I want to hear from you about anything else you want to talk to me about, too."

Learn to receive. Many people find this to be embarrassing, and question whether they deserve what their loved ones want to give. How can we learn to receive? Sometimes cancer forces the issue. For example, when you just cannot do the things necessary for your own well being, you have to ask for help. Other times, you can ease into it, intentionally receiving a bit, then more (like having a friend take your children to soccer practices). Ask yourself: would your loved ones deserve to receive help and care from you, were your circumstances reversed? Then why not you? Consider this: how would you feel if they refused your offer of help? Cancer, thankfully, has a way of severely disrupting the perfectionist standards many of us learned in childhood.

Depend on your loved ones. They want you to. Let them know what you'd like them to do for you. You could even ask them to do something you would do if you could for someone else. One woman had her sister tell their mother about the recurrence so that she would not have to see the look on her mother's face. That way she didn't have to bear the full load of disclosing the bad news. Avoid expressing your gratitude constantly, in a guilty way. Let yourself receive. One heartfelt thank you is enough.

One of the ways people stay balanced while living with cancer is to imagine their hands held open before them, one holding the reality "I might live. I just might live." The other hand holds the reality "This cancer might take my life long before I ever thought I'd die." Those who grasp only the possibility of living can become very anxious, for the opposite reality is also possible. Those who grasp only the possibility of dying sooner than they hoped can become stuck in depression. Hold both possibilities, lightly if you can, and remember: the weights in your hands will fluctuate, back and forth. The days you feel dispirited and down won't last. The days you feel filled with hope and confident you'll do well won't either. Remember the cancer motto: "Right now I'm OK. If that changes I'll deal with it, because that's what I do."

Consider joining a cancer support group. Although you are unique in your experience of cancer, the other group members are the only people who can come close to really understanding how you feel. Many cancer centers provide support for caregivers, too.

If you're not drawn to a support group, you can ask one of your medical providers, like your oncologist, a nurse, or the oncology counselor to contact another person with breast cancer and ask if he or she would be willing to contact you. Many people going through or finishing treatment themselves volunteer to call others who could use a listening ear. These relationships can become special and powerful sources of support, encouragement, and understanding.

Consider starting a fear journal that you write in for only 15-20 minutes at a time, perhaps daily, or when you feel the need. Pour your fears into it and then close it, leaving them there. Don't read and re-read it. Let them stay there. You might also start a list of things you'd like to do for the next week, month, or the next year. These aren't plans, but hopes. Planning for only a short time ahead can remind you of living well in spite of cancer and prevent you from feeling overwhelmed or uncomfortable.

Having cancer is a lonely experience. You probably feel alone, even if you are embraced by an entire group of people who love you, added to an excellent team of medical professionals, along with even the prayers of strangers. This is a time when you will learn to love and care for yourself in new ways. You will find strengths and resilience, paths to peace and rest, because cancer will teach you these things. This you can trust.

If you are a woman who has struggled with sexual abuse or assault in the past, it is normal to feel those feelings all over again when you endure the invasive experience of treatment for breast cancer. If you have not already done so, seek a counselor who can help you manage your feelings, supporting and guiding you toward the deep wisdom and acceptance that working through such hurts can generate. This process of supported healing can help you come to terms with the losses caused by assault so that you can think of them without the hurt and difficult feelings that you have lived with for so long. A kind, loving and skilled therapist who can help you with emotional exploration and expression will provide the most effective assistance. If you are in crisis, a therapist also trained in EFT (Emotional Freedom Techniques) or EMDR (Eye Movement Desensitization and Reprocessing) can help you learn to calm your anxiety quickly.

If you are a man with breast cancer, as 1% of breast cancer survivors are, you may carry the added burden of embarrassment at having what many consider to be a woman's disease. You may not be welcome at women's breast cancer support groups where a lot of "show and tell" happens. However, your needs for support are just as important. The cancer center may offer a general cancer support group you could attend. People there will understand and have your back.

Feeling embarrassed about hair loss or looking as exhausted as you feel can be very hard. When friends ask if there is something they can do for you, you might suggest they take you to buy a beautiful scarf, or take you to consult with a make-up specialist. You could suggest a scarf party be held for you. Have the organizer suggest people buy only soft, cotton scarves for you, since they won't slip on your head when your hair is gone. You may feel more at peace with your appearance if you surrender to it and find ways to kindly see yourself through the long walk of hair re-growth and energy renewal, replacing critical self-talk with kindness and acceptance, in soft and loving tones.

Sexuality. So many women struggling with side effects

from treatment are upset about the sudden and what feels like permanent, irrevocable disappearance of their sexual feelings. Feelings of guilt can exist for both partners, one for not wanting to make love, the other for wanting to. Talk together about ways that are comfortable and meaningful to physically express your love. The spontaneity of love-making can feel lost, but remember when you first began your sexual relationship? For many, there was nothing spontaneous about it. You spent time and effort preparing, lighting candles, choosing what to wear, selecting special music. When cancer treatment is done, your sexual feelings may well return, and for many couples, getting through such a crisis together has strengthened their relationship so that love making becomes an even deeper, more loving experience than it was before.

Beware of something that might called "the positive trap". No doubt you have heard the well-meaning advice, "Be positive!", many times, in many ways. People with cancer fear that if they are not thinking positively they will not get well, and might even die. But the opposite is true. Research shows that holding in the "negative" feelings such as anxiety, anger or sadness can be harmful to immune function in an indirect way. Expression of emotions—all of them—is an important part of staying healthy throughout the cancer journey. It is important to know someone who can listen to all of your emotions, hopeful and not, without imparting judgment or fear. By expressing them, you can let the scary feelings go and learn to take one day, or even one moment, at a time. Remember this cancer motto: "In this moment I am OK. If that changes I'll deal with it, because that's what I do." Tape this to a place where you will see it every day. Remember it. It's true.

People express emotions in a variety of ways. You may need to cry or you may feel relieved simply to acknowledge or describe your feelings of sadness. Men and women are often different in this way. No one way is better than another.

There are other benefits of expressing your fears, anger and sadness with someone you trust. When you do, hope that was hidden under those feelings bubbles up to the surface of your awareness. Expressing fears frees the hope to rise.

Sometimes people with cancer feel their hopes have died. Hopes that cannot be realized die, but new hopes always wait in the wings for us to discover them. What are you hoping for today? Make a list of your hopes, the ones that will make today better, and the big ones you hope to be fulfilled down the road. Review your list frequently, revise it, and share it with someone you're close to. This can lighten your spirit, and help define what you choose to do with the energy you have to use today.

When you become most discouraged, call a meeting with your closest friends and ask them to tell you why they want you to live. Allow their words to sink into you, encourage you, give you comfort, and inspire you.

Consider asking your care team for a referral to an oncology family therapist or counselor who can see you individually or include your family and other loved ones. Such a person can explore ways of coping that will work for you and help you all manage the many, sometimes conflicting ways people cope with their fear of losing someone they love and depend upon.

As we have seen, an experience of cancer changes people and the lives they are living. When it comes to managing your life after cancer, when treatment is completed, it can help to redefine your whole life, as daunting as that sounds. Take adequate time to think, write, and talk about what your "new normal" life looks like, exploring this idea as it relates to your body (what you can do to keep it well), your mind (how you are thinking differently about your life, what thoughts sustain you and nourish you now), your heart (how you take care of yourself emotionally when you fear a recurrence, and how you let others love you in new ways now), and your spirit (how you think and feel differently about God and spirituality in your life after treatment is done). A "new normal" life is made up of what has changed because

Nurse's Note:

It is important for you to be comfortable with your care team. This is just as important to them as it is to you.

26

of the cancer, and includes what you have lost as a result of cancer, what you have gained as a result of cancer, what you are choosing to let go of as a result of cancer, and what you are choosing to let in now, as a result of cancer.

Chapter Five

Focusing On Your Spirit

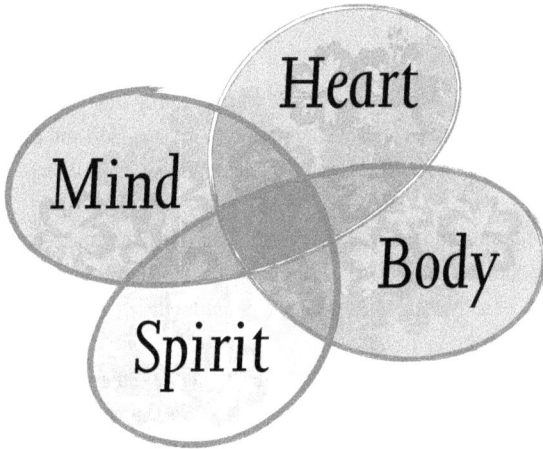

Heart

Mind

Body

Spirit

**The Ways You Think And Feel About God
And Your Spirituality**

"Why did God give me this cancer?"

"Breast cancer blew my spirit open. It made me embrace what I already knew, but be it and think it more, thankfully. I know I'm not alone, ever."

"I've never been religious or spiritual. It was never part of my upbringing. But I don't know where to turn to inside myself now."

"What can I count on and control? The love I give and receive. I can take that for granted when everything else is falling apart."

"Before, I was angry at God for my early life. I stopped being angry at God when I got cancer."

"Cancer is like the holocaust, or the tsunami. God wasn't mad at all those people who died."

"I get restless in church for the first time in my life. I used to love it. It feels meaningless to me now, and I don't know why. That scares me. I've lost God."

"My mind likes to take control, and then connection to my spirit feels lost. Cancer has forced me inside, into this moment. Then I can find myself again."

"It's awful. My life was focused on my healthy lifestyle. I felt invincible. Cancer can happen anyway, to anyone. How can anybody feel safe, ever? If this can happen, anything can go wrong."

"My grandmother used to tell me, 'Security is knowing that we have none, except for God'. It confused me, but I never forgot. I think I finally understand what she meant by that."

"I'm still looking for spiritual tools. I want a connection with God on a more consistent basis, every day. No matter what I'm facing I want to have a sense of peace about it. I pray for peace."

"When I'm scared I'm trying to lean toward my wisdom instead of my fear."

"Cancer has helped me spiritually. I liked things to be the way I wanted them to be, before. Now I can let things just be the way they are. It's a more peaceful way to live. I could never figure out how to be this way, until now."

"I envy my friends who have what they call 'faith'. When there is nowhere to look, where do I look?"

"I learned how to fight, and hang on, and find solutions along the way. But now I'm told it's time to call Hospice. How can I let go of all I've learned and let myself die?"

"If I don't stop trying to control what I can't control—the cancer—and resent it, and be angry at it, I'll never heal into the kind of person I want to become. I want something good to come out of this whether I make it out alive or not."

"I'm trying to forgive myself for wasting the gifts I was given in this life. I could have done more, made more of an impact."

"I learned very well to get through years of cancer fears by living one day at a time, looking only at the small picture of what was immediately demanded of me. Now it seems I have to say goodbye and look at the big picture again. That is hard to do. Where am I going?"

"My wife and I look at the circle of life. Dying goes on every minute of every day, everywhere. It's normal and natural. It's easy to see that in nature. That comforts me."

Tips For The Journey:

In our lives, we all face three sets of lessons that teach us wisdom: the lessons of the dark (learning to let go of thoughts and beliefs that no longer fit or are hurtful to ourselves, and learning to feel whole in solitude), lessons of light (learning to let love in and hold on to it, walking through the fire that burns away our defenses, allowing for the depth and joy of emotional and spiritual intimacy) and lessons of the gray (learning to simply wait when we have already leaped into mid-air, relinquishing what no longer works well, but haven't yet landed at the next level of understanding or peace. This is practicing spiritual patience, and it's one of the most difficult tasks of all.)

It is common for people who are facing a trauma or crisis with no quick resolution to feel lost in the wilderness of their experience, beyond the reach of God. This can happen even as belief in God and in the power of God's love remain clear and strong. The feelings of loss and the impulse to justify the loss with thoughts of cancer as punishment can be devastating. What may be true instead is that when we fall off a cliff, so to speak, and are in a deeper, darker place than we've ever known, we need to do the important work of allowing God to find us. God seeks us, just as we seek God. Again, this can be a time of waiting, and the work is learning spiritual patience.

Many people do not consider themselves religious, or even spiritual. If this is true for you, it might help to define, clarify and focus on which values mean the most to you, and the beliefs that have sustained you throughout your life. How have you used these values to guide your choices during difficult experiences in the past? What have you learned about yourself having survived past crises? What gives your life meaning now? Where do you find hope now?

If the idea of faith is new and appealing, talk with people whose faith you admire, whose faith guides the choices they make. Let them be the first of many teachers.

When you feel most afraid or disheartened, what do you need to remember? What spiritual beliefs can you lean into now? Close your eyes and softly allow them to hold you, surround you, and fill you with peace. Allow all of the stress and anxiety to flow through you, going on its way without you. Become the boulder in the river of fear.

What are you praying for? Many people find their prayers changing as they move through the experience of cancer. From prayers of pleading and longing, based upon fears, they find themselves simply asking for strength to move to the next step, trust to help manage fear, or the wisdom to allow the journey to take the path it needs to take, and the time it requires. Some simply ask for help.

Do you pray for yourself? Many people do not, and consider doing so to be selfish. Yet, when it comes to our spiritual health, we need to ask for what we want, and open to the answers as they come. You may become more comfortable seeking on your own behalf if you allow yourself to ask for qualities you need to be able to grow spiritually through the experience of cancer. For example: "Please help me to always feel Your presence in my heart...teach me to feel the peace I know is there, waiting behind my fears...fill me with trust in those who are working to make me better...give me patience and tolerance to bear this vulnerability...". Then you need to become aware of these qualities coming alive inside you. Asking is only half of the process.

Some say that prayer is speaking with God, while meditation is listening to God. You might decide to meditate. Mindfulness Meditation, practiced daily for 8 weeks, has been shown on MRIs to increase the amount of brain matter in the part of the brain where we manage fears. Such a practice trains our brains to let go of frightening thoughts, so they are no longer as capable of "kidnapping" our minds. Meditation teaches us to bring our attention to the present moment, when our lives can feel safe. It is fore thoughts of loss that cause us to worry.

When it comes time to die, we prepare ourselves. Hospice workers consistently hear patients say things that reflect a growing peace about letting go of this precious life, beloved families and loved ones, and work left unfinished. We somehow come to understand, when it is time to move on, that we have left enough of a legacy behind, that the energy of our passion for life is palpable and available for those we are leaving, and it is enough. How can this happen? Perhaps it is because we finally learn that being, when we can no longer do, illuminates an enhancement of our life energy, not a diminishment.

In Summary...

Learning to live and thrive with breast cancer requires that you focus on all the parts of your life—how you act, how you think, how you feel, and how you let yourself be loved—

so that you can flow through this life altering experience, and arrive at a better place afterward, knowing your ability to heal and your own wholeness more deeply than you ever knew them before. For your body: rest, exercise, massage (with an oncology trained massage therapist), guided imagery (which is a journey inside your mind which can positively impact your body) yoga, acupuncture, relaxing breathing techniques and other complementary services can help. For your mind: cognitive behavioral therapy, family therapy, and seeking the guidance of those who have walked this path before you can diminish much of the stress. For your heart: emotional support, learning to cast a loving eye on yourself, family therapy, and seeking the wisdom of the wisest people you know, and the guidance of those who have been there, can help create your new path. For your spirit: prayer, consultations with spiritual teachers, developing a meditation practice, and silent retreats may illuminate the way ahead.

Because of the cancer, you and the people you love have been forced to consider the possibility of your death earlier than any of you would have thought necessary. As difficult and frightening as this is, it is also a gift. As you consider coming to terms with dying, you gain the wisdom of this journey earlier, and it can have an intentional positive impact on your own future and on the future of everyone who loves you. However you choose to move forward, encouraging yourself to fight the cancer and not yourself, and allowing yourself to receive in all of the ways mentioned above, will make a difference in both the quality of your journey now, and the feelings of peace which await.

Resources:

Kitchen Table Wisdom: Stories that Heal by Rachel Naomi Remen MD

The Anxiety and Phobia Workbook by Edmund Bourne PhD

Comfortable With Uncertainty by Pema Chodron

Grace For Each Hour: Through The Breast Cancer Journey by Mary J. Nelson

The Places That Scare You by Pema Chodron

The Wisdom of No Escape by Pema Chodron

Final Gifts by Maggie Callanan and Patricia Kelley

Internet Resources:

healthjourneys.com for powerful, tested, guided imagery CDs. Use your mind to impact your body in helpful ways.

wellspouse.org

American Cancer Society

Inspire.com

caringbridge.com

helpinghands.com

pandora.com (radio): Calm Meditation music

For Children:

Help Me Say Goodbye: Activities for Helping Kids Cope When a Special Person Dies

Nana Upstairs, Nana Downstairs by Tomi dePaola

Tear Soup by Schwiebert, DeKlyen, and Bills

The Hope Tree by Laura Numeroff and Wendy S. Harpham MD

Journal

Journal

Common Cancer Terms

Adenocarcinoma: Cancer that originates from the glandular tissue of the breast.

Adjuvant therapy: Treatment used in addition to the main form of therapy. It usually refers to treatment utilized after surgery. As an example, chemotherapy or radiation may be given after surgery to increase the chance of cure.

Angiogenesis: The process of forming new blood vessels. Some cancer therapies work by blocking angiogenesis, and this blocks nutrients from reaching cancer cells.

Antigen: A substance that triggers an immune response by the body. This immune response involves the body making antibodies.

Benign tumor: An abnormal growth that is not cancer and does not spread to other areas of the body.

Biopsy: The removal of a sample of tissue to detect whether cancer is present.

Brachytherapy: Internal radiation treatment given by placing radioactive seeds or pellets directly in the tumor or next to it.

Cancer: The process of cells growing out of control due to mutations in DNA.

Carcinoma: A malignant tumor (cancer) that starts in the lining layer of organs. The most frequent types are lung, breast, colon, and prostate.

Chemotherapy: Medicine usually given by an IV or in pill form to stop cancer cells from dividing and spreading.

Clinical Trials: Research studies that allow testing of new treatments or drugs and compare the outcomes to standard treatments. Before the new treatment is studied on patients, it is studied in the laboratory. The human studies are called clinical trials.

Computerized Axial Tomography: Otherwise known as a CT scan. This is a picture taken to evaluate the anatomy of the body in three dimensions.

Cytokine: A product of the immune system that may stimulate immunity and cause shrinkage of some cancers.

Deoxyribonucleic Acid: Otherwise known as DNA. The genetic blueprint found in the nucleus of the cell. The DNA holds information on cell growth, division, and function.

Enzyme: A protein that increases the rate of chemical reactions in living cells.

Feeding tube: A flexible tube placed in the stomach through which nutrition can be given.

Gastro Esophageal Reflux Disease (GERD): A condition in which stomach acid moves up into the esophagus and causes a burning sensation.

Genetic Testing: Tests performed to determine whether someone has certain genes which increase cancer risk.

Grade: A measurement of how abnormal a cell looks under a microscope. Cancers with more abnormal appearing cells (higher grade tumors) have the tendency to be faster growing and have a worse prognosis.

Hereditary Cancer Syndrome: Conditions that are associated with cancer development and can occur in family members because of a mutated gene.

Histology: A description of the cancer cells which can distinguish what part of the body the cells originated from.

Immunotherapy: Treatments that promote or support the body's immune system response to a disease such as cancer.

Intensity Modulated Radiation Therapy: Also known as IMRT. A complex type of radiation therapy where many beams are used. It spares surrounding normal tissues and treats the cancer with more precision.

Leukemia: Cancer of the blood or blood-forming organs. People with leukemia often have a noticeable increase in white blood cells (leukocytes).

Localized cancer: Cancer that has not spread to another part of the body.

Lymph nodes: Bean shaped structures that are the "filter" of the body. The fluid that passes through them is called lymph fluid and filters unwanted materials like cancer cells, bacteria, and viruses.

Malignant: A tumor that is cancer.

Metastasis: The spread of cancer cells to other parts of the body such as the lungs or bones.

Monoclonal Antibodies: Antibodies made in the lab to work as homing devices for cancer cells.

Mutation: A change in the DNA of a cell. Cancer is caused by mutations in the cell which lead to abnormal growth and function of the cell.

Neoadjuvant therapy: Systemic and/or radiation treatment given before surgery to shrink a tumor.

Palliative treatment: Treatment that relieves symptoms, such as pain, but is not expected to cure the disease. Its main purpose is to improve the patient's quality of life.

Pathologist: A doctor trained to recognize tumor cells as benign or cancerous.

Positron Emission Tomography: Also known as a PET scan. This test is used to look at cell metabolism to recognize areas in the body where the cancer may be hiding.

Radiation therapy: Invisible high energy beams that can shrink or kill cancer cells.

Recurrence: When cancer comes back after treatment.

Remission: Partial or complete disappearance of the signs and symptoms of cancer. This is not necessarily a cure.

Risk factors: Environmental and genetic factors that increase our chance of getting cancer.

Side effects: Unwanted effects of treatment such as hair loss, burns or rash on the skin, sore throat, etc.

Simulation: Mapping session where radiation is planned. If the doctor will be using a mask for your treatment, this is the time it will be custom fit for your face.

Staging: Tests that help to determine if the cancer has spread to lymph nodes or other organs.

Standard Therapy: The most commonly used and widely accepted form of treatment that has been tested and proven.

Targeted Therapy: Modern cancer treatments that attack the part of cancer cells that make them different from normal cells. Targeted agents tend to have different side effects than conventional chemotherapy drugs.

Tumor: A new growth of tissue which forms a lump on or inside the body that may or may not be cancerous.

About The Authors

Tess Taft, MSW, LICSW: Tess is an oncology stress management specialist and family therapist who has served cancer patients and their loved ones in hospitals, cancer clinics, homes, nursing homes, hospices and private practice settings for 34 years. She received a Masters Degree in Social Work from The University of Washington in 1979 and completed a Marriage and Family Therapy training program in 1981. In 1990 she became a certified specialist in Interactive Guided Imagery for Medical Clinicians in order to teach clients this unique and powerful tool to help with symptom and stress management, and to explore and deepen hope and faith. She has taught a Palliative Care certification program for graduate social work students at Eastern Washington University since 2007, which includes 3 classes: Family Systems and Illness, Death and Dying, and Alternatives in Healing. Tess has provided trainings nationally, as well as clinical supervision for many therapists over the years. She is committed to serving people whose life-threatening diagnosis, or that of a love, has propelled them on a journey inside themselves to find emotional and spiritual healing and peace.

Kathy Beach, RN: Kathy graduated with her RN degree in 1993. She decided to get a degree in nursing after her mother was diagnosed with breast cancer. She spent sixteen years in hospital nursing where she worked on a wide range of units from Medical Oncology to Outpatient Surgery. For the past 4 years, she has focused her energy in oncology and radiation oncology with Cancer Care Northwest in Spokane, WA. She loves her work and finds the patients she cares for and their families to be extremely inspiring.

Christopher M. Lee, MD: Dr. Lee is a practicing Radiation Oncologist and is the Director of Research for Cancer Care Northwest and The

Gamma Knife of Spokane (Spokane, WA). Dr. Lee graduated cum laude in Biochemistry from Brigham Young University in 1997 which included a summer research fellowship at Harvard University and Brigham and Women's Hospital. He subsequently attended Saint Louis University School of Medicine where he received his M.D. with Distinction in Research degree. He completed four additional years of specialty training in Radiation Oncology at the Huntsman Cancer Hospital and University of Utah Medical Center during which he was given multiple national awards. Dr. Lee has actively pursued both basic science and clinical research throughout his career. He continues to be a proliferative author of scientific papers and regularly gives presentations on radiotherapy technique and the use of targeted radiation in the care of patients with head and neck (throat), brain, breast, gynecologic, and prostate malignancies.

www.ingramcontent.com/pod-product-compliance
Lightning Source LLC
Chambersburg PA
CBHW071103040426
42443CB00013B/3390